MAXWELL THOMAS

10 Weight Loss Hacks For Men Over 40

Ten simple ways for men aged 40 and over to lose weight

Contents

Introduction

Welcome to 10 Weight Loss Hacks For Men Aged Over 40. Losing weight can be a challenging process, especially as we age. As men age, their metabolism slows down and they tend to lose muscle mass. This can make it more difficult to lose weight, as the body burns fewer calories at rest. Hormonal changes can also play a role, as testosterone levels tend to decline with age, which can lead to an increase in body fat.

Additionally, lifestyle factors such as a sedentary lifestyle, poor diet, and lack of sleep can contribute to weight gain and make it more difficult to lose weight. However, there are many strategies that men over 40 can use to lose weight, such as drinking more water, eating more protein, getting enough sleep, reducing sugar intake, and exercising regularly.

In this book, we will discuss 10 weight loss hacks that can help you achieve your goals. By making these simple changes to their diet and lifestyle, men over 40 can achieve and maintain a healthy weight.

Hack 1 - Drink More Water

Drinking water can be an effective tool for weight loss. One of the primary ways that water can help with weight loss is by increasing feelings of fullness and reducing hunger. Drinking water before meals can help to fill the stomach and reduce the amount of food that is consumed, leading to a reduction in overall calorie intake. Additionally, thirst can often be mistaken for hunger, so drinking water can help to prevent overeating.

Another way that water can help with weight loss is by increasing calorie burning. Drinking water can help to boost the metabolism, which can lead to an increase in calorie burning. Additionally, drinking cold water can help to burn more calories, as the body has to work harder to warm up the water to body temperature.

Drinking water can also help to remove waste from the body, which can contribute to weight loss. When the body is dehydrated, it cannot properly remove waste as urine or feces. Water helps the kidneys to filter toxins and waste while retaining essential nutrients and electrolytes. When the body is dehydrated, the kidneys retain fluid, which can lead to bloating and water retention. Drinking water can help to keep waste moving by softening or loosening hardened stools, which can help to prevent constipation and bloating.

Finally, drinking water can help to reduce liquid calorie intake. Sugary drinks like soda and juice are high in calories and can contribute to weight gain. By swapping sugary drinks for water, individuals can cut down on empty calories and reduce their overall calorie intake.

In conclusion, drinking water can be an effective tool for weight loss. By increasing feelings of fullness, boosting calorie burning, removing waste from the body, and reducing liquid calorie intake, water can help individuals achieve and maintain a healthy weight.

Here are some ideas to help with increasing water intake:

Carry a water bottle:
   Carrying a water bottle with you throughout the day can help you stay hydrated and make it easier to drink water regularly.

Eat water-rich foods:
   Foods such as cucumbers, watermelon, lettuce, strawberries, tomatoes, and celery are high in water content and can help you stay hydrated.

Drink water before meals:
   Drinking water before meals can help you feel fuller and reduce your calorie intake.

Drink water instead of sugary drinks:
   Sugary drinks such as soda, juice, and sports drinks can be high in calories and sugar. Drinking water instead can help you reduce your calorie intake and stay hydrated. If you find plain water unappetizing, try using water enhancers, opting for pre-flavored waters, serving fruit juice diluted with water, or making infused waters.

Set reminders:

Setting reminders on your phone or computer can help you remember to drink water throughout the day.

Hack 2 - Eat More Protein

Eating protein can be an effective tool for weight loss. One of the primary ways that protein can help with weight loss is by increasing feelings of fullness and reducing hunger. Protein is more filling than carbohydrates or fat, so adding more protein to your diet can help you feel full and reduce your overall calorie intake. Additionally, protein takes longer to digest than carbohydrates or fat, which means that it stays in your stomach longer and helps you feel full for a longer period of time.

Another way that protein can help with weight loss is by increasing calorie burning. Protein has a higher thermic effect than carbohydrates or fat, which means that the body burns more calories digesting protein than it does digesting carbohydrates or fat. Additionally, protein can help to preserve muscle mass during weight loss, which can help to increase calorie burning and prevent weight regain.

Protein can also help to reduce cravings and prevent overeating. Eating protein can help to stabilize blood sugar levels, which can help to reduce cravings for sugary or high-carbohydrate foods. Additionally, protein can help to reduce the production of ghrelin, a hormone that stimulates appetite, which can help to reduce hunger and prevent overeating.

Finally, protein can help to reduce body fat and increase lean muscle mass. Eating protein can help to increase muscle protein synthesis, which is the process by which the body builds new muscle tissue. Additionally, protein can help to reduce body fat by increasing the body's metabolic rate and promoting fat burning.

In conclusion, eating protein can be an effective tool for weight loss. By increasing feelings of fullness, boosting calorie burning, reducing cravings, and increasing lean muscle mass, protein can help individuals achieve and maintain a healthy weight.

Here are some ideas to help with increasing protein intake:

Add sauces and seasonings:
   Research shows that the taste and flavor of high-protein foods can encourage older adults to consume more of them. Adding sauces and seasonings to meals can increase the consumption of high-protein foods.

Add cheese, nuts or seeds:
   Cheese, nuts, and seeds are naturally high in protein and can be added to meals to increase protein intake. Cheese can be easily added to soups, salads, pasta, or mashed potatoes. Nuts and seeds can be added to breakfast cereals, salads, and desserts such as yogurts.

Eat eggs for breakfast:
   Eggs are a great source of protein and can be easily incorporated into breakfast meals to boost protein intake.

Choose protein-rich snacks:
   Snacks such as jerky, hard-boiled eggs, and Greek yogurt are high in

protein and can help increase protein intake.

Choose protein-rich foods:

Foods such as beef, chicken, fish, eggs, milk, cheese, nuts, and beans are rich in protein and can help you meet your daily protein requirements.

Hack 3 – Get Enough Sleep

Getting enough sleep is an important factor in maintaining a healthy weight. Lack of sleep can lead to weight gain and obesity, as well as other health problems such as diabetes and heart disease. There are several ways in which getting enough sleep can help with weight loss.

One way that sleep can help with weight loss is by regulating hormones that control appetite. Lack of sleep can lead to an increase in the hormone ghrelin, which stimulates appetite, and a decrease in the hormone leptin, which signals fullness. This can lead to overeating and weight gain. Getting enough sleep can help to regulate these hormones and reduce appetite, which can lead to weight loss.

Another way that sleep can help with weight loss is by reducing stress. Lack of sleep can lead to an increase in the stress hormone cortisol, which can lead to weight gain and other health problems. Getting enough sleep can help to reduce stress and lower cortisol levels, which can lead to weight loss.

Sleep can also help to increase energy levels and improve exercise performance. Lack of sleep can lead to fatigue and reduced motivation to exercise, which can lead to weight gain. Getting enough sleep can help to increase energy levels and improve exercise performance, which can lead to weight loss.

Finally, getting enough sleep can help to reduce late-night snacking. Lack of sleep can lead to an increase in cravings for high-calorie, high-carbohydrate foods, which can lead to overeating and weight gain. Getting enough sleep can help to reduce these cravings and prevent late-night snacking, which can lead to weight loss.

In conclusion, getting enough sleep is an important factor in maintaining a healthy weight. By regulating hormones that control appetite, reducing stress, increasing energy levels, and reducing late-night snacking, sleep can help individuals achieve and maintain a healthy weight.

Here are some ideas to help with getting enough sleep:

Establish a regular sleep schedule:
   Going to bed and waking up at the same time every day can help regulate your body's internal clock and improve the quality of your sleep.

Create a relaxing bedtime routine:
   A relaxing bedtime routine can help you unwind and prepare for sleep. This could include taking a warm bath, reading a book, or listening to calming music.

Exercise during the day:
   Regular exercise can help you fall asleep faster and improve the quality of your sleep.

Avoid caffeine and alcohol at night:
   Caffeine and alcohol can interfere with your sleep cycle, making it

harder to fall asleep and stay asleep.

Create a sleep-friendly environment:

Make sure your bedroom is cool, dark, and quiet. Use comfortable bedding and pillows, and avoid using electronic devices before bedtime.

Hack 4 – Reduce Sugar Intake

Reducing sugar intake can be an effective tool for weight loss. One of the primary ways that reducing sugar intake can help with weight loss is by reducing overall calorie intake. Sugary foods and drinks are often high in calories and can contribute to weight gain. By reducing sugar intake, individuals can reduce their overall calorie intake and create a calorie deficit, which can lead to weight loss.

Another way that reducing sugar intake can help with weight loss is by reducing cravings for sugary foods. Sugar can be addictive, and consuming sugary foods and drinks can lead to cravings for more sugar. By reducing sugar intake, individuals can reduce their cravings for sugary foods and drinks, which can help them to make healthier food choices and reduce their overall calorie intake.

Reducing sugar intake can also help to reduce inflammation in the body. Consuming too much sugar can lead to chronic inflammation, which can contribute to a variety of health problems, including obesity. By reducing sugar intake, individuals can reduce inflammation in the body, which can help to promote weight loss and improve overall health.

Finally, reducing sugar intake can help to improve insulin sensitivity. Consuming too much sugar can lead to insulin resistance, which can contribute to weight gain and other health problems. By reducing sugar intake, individuals can improve insulin sensitivity, which can help to promote weight loss and reduce the risk of developing type 2 diabetes.

In conclusion, reducing sugar intake can be an effective tool for weight loss. By reducing overall calorie intake, reducing cravings for sugary foods, reducing inflammation in the body, and improving insulin sensitivity, reducing sugar intake can help individuals achieve and maintain a healthy weight.

Here are some ideas to help with reducing sugar intake:

Choose whole foods:
   Avoid highly processed foods and choose whole foods instead. This can help you reduce your sugar intake and improve your overall health.

Read food labels:
   Food labels tell you how much sugar a food contains. Look for foods that are low in sugar and avoid those that are high in sugar.

Drink water:
   Choose water over sugary drinks like fizzy soda, cordial, or fruit juice. If you find plain water unappetizing, try using water enhancers, opting for pre-flavored waters, serving fruit juice diluted with water, or making infused waters.

Choose low-calorie sweeteners:
   Some individuals can achieve some success by reducing consumption of added sugars by choosing foods and beverages sweetened with low- and no-calorie sweeteners (LNCS) and using their preferred type and forms of table-top LNCS to sweeten foods and beverages.

Avoid processed foods:

Processed foods often contain added sugars. Choosing whole foods instead can help you reduce your sugar intake.

Hack 5 – Eat More Fiber

Eating more fiber can be an effective tool for weight loss. One of the primary ways that fiber can help with weight loss is by increasing feelings of fullness and reducing hunger. Fiber is a type of carbohydrate that cannot be digested by the body, so it passes through the digestive system relatively unchanged. This means that it takes up space in the stomach and helps to create a feeling of fullness, which can reduce overall calorie intake.

Another way that fiber can help with weight loss is by slowing down the absorption of carbohydrates. When carbohydrates are consumed, they are broken down into simple sugars and absorbed into the bloodstream. This can cause a rapid increase in blood sugar levels, which can lead to an increase in insulin production and a subsequent drop in blood sugar levels. This can cause hunger and cravings for more carbohydrates. By slowing down the absorption of carbohydrates, fiber can help to regulate blood sugar levels and reduce hunger and cravings.

Fiber can also help to reduce the number of calories that are absorbed by the body. When fiber is consumed, it binds to other nutrients in the digestive system, such as fat and sugar, and helps to prevent their absorption into the bloodstream. This can lead to a reduction in overall calorie intake and can contribute to weight loss.

Finally, fiber can help to promote the growth of healthy gut bacteria. The gut microbiome plays an important role in overall health, including weight management. Studies have shown that individuals with a more diverse gut microbiome tend to be leaner than those with a less diverse microbiome. Fiber can help to promote the growth of healthy gut bacteria, which can lead to improved gut health and weight loss.

In conclusion, eating more fiber can be an effective tool for weight loss. By increasing feelings of fullness, slowing down the absorption of carbohydrates, reducing the number of calories absorbed by the body, and promoting the growth of healthy gut bacteria, fiber can help individuals achieve and maintain a healthy weight.

Here are some ideas to help with eating more fiber:

Choose whole foods:
   Whole foods such as fruits, vegetables, whole grains, and legumes are rich in fiber and can help you meet your daily fiber requirements.

Read food labels:
   Food labels tell you how much fiber a food contains. Look for foods that are high in fiber and avoid those that are low in fiber.

Add fiber-rich foods to your diet:
   Add fiber-rich foods such as chia seeds, flaxseeds, and psyllium husk to your diet. These foods are high in fiber and can help you meet your daily fiber requirements.

Gradually increase your fiber intake:
   Gradually increase your fiber intake over a few weeks to allow your digestive system to adjust to the change. Also, drink plenty of water,

as fiber works best when it absorbs water, making your stool soft and bulky.

Choose high-fiber snacks:
Snacks such as nuts, seeds, and fruit are rich in fiber and can help you meet your daily fiber requirements.

Hack 6 – Reduce Your Stress Levels

Reducing stress levels can be an effective tool for weight loss. One of the primary ways that reducing stress levels can help with weight loss is by reducing cortisol levels. Cortisol is a hormone that is released in response to stress, and it can lead to an increase in appetite and weight gain. By reducing stress levels, individuals can reduce cortisol levels and prevent overeating, which can lead to weight loss.

Another way that reducing stress levels can help with weight loss is by improving sleep quality. Stress can disrupt sleep patterns and lead to poor sleep quality, which can contribute to weight gain. By reducing stress levels, individuals can improve sleep quality and promote weight loss.

Reducing stress levels can also help to reduce emotional eating. Many people turn to food as a way to cope with stress, which can lead to overeating and weight gain. By reducing stress levels, individuals can reduce emotional eating and make healthier food choices, which can lead to weight loss.

Finally, reducing stress levels can help to improve exercise performance. Stress can lead to fatigue and reduced motivation to exercise, which can lead to weight gain. By reducing stress levels, individuals can increase energy levels and improve exercise performance, which can lead to weight loss.

In conclusion, reducing stress levels can be an effective tool for weight loss. By reducing cortisol levels, improving sleep quality, reducing emotional eating, and improving exercise performance, reducing stress levels can help individuals achieve and maintain a healthy weight.

Here are some ideas to help with reducing stress levels:

Exercise regularly:

Regular exercise can help you reduce stress levels and improve your overall health.

Practice relaxation techniques:

Relaxation techniques such as yoga, tai chi, meditation, guided imagery, and deep breathing exercises can help you elicit the relaxation response, which helps lower blood pressure, heart rate, breathing rate, oxygen consumption, and stress hormones.

Get enough sleep:

Establishing "sleep-friendly" routines can help reduce stress-related insomnia and other negative effects. Sleep quality can be improved with a comfortable mattress that fits your sleep preferences.

Socialize:

Socializing with friends and family can help you reduce stress levels and improve your overall well-being.

Eat a healthy diet:

Eating a healthy diet can help you reduce stress levels and improve your overall health.

19

Hack 7 – Exercise Regularly

Regular exercise can be an effective tool for weight loss. One of the primary ways that exercise can help with weight loss is by burning calories. When the body burns more calories than it consumes, it creates a calorie deficit, which can lead to weight loss. Additionally, exercise can help to increase muscle mass, which can lead to an increase in calorie burning and weight loss.

Another way that exercise can help with weight loss is by reducing appetite. Exercise can help to regulate hormones that control appetite, such as ghrelin and leptin, which can lead to a reduction in overall calorie intake. Additionally, exercise can help to reduce cravings for high-calorie, high-carbohydrate foods, which can lead to overeating and weight gain.

Exercise can also help to reduce stress, which can contribute to weight gain. Stress can lead to an increase in the hormone cortisol, which can lead to an increase in appetite and weight gain. Exercise can help to reduce cortisol levels and promote weight loss.

Finally, exercise can help to improve sleep quality. Poor sleep quality can lead to weight gain and obesity, as well as other health problems such as diabetes and heart disease. Exercise can help to improve sleep quality and promote weight loss.

In conclusion, regular exercise can be an effective tool for weight loss. By burning calories, increasing muscle mass, reducing appetite, reducing stress, and improving sleep quality, exercise can help individuals achieve and maintain a healthy weight.

Here are some ideas to help with getting regular exercise:

High-Intensity Interval Training (HIIT):
HIIT workouts alternate short bursts of high intensity (maximum effort) with periods of low intensity (active rest). It has been scientifically proven to increase metabolic rate and improve heart health.

Strength training:
Strength training can help you build muscle mass, increase bone density, and improve balance and coordination. Some key strength training exercises for men over 40 include squats, deadlifts, bench press, overhead press, bent-over rows, pull-ups, and planks.

Flexibility and mobility exercises:
Flexibility and mobility exercises such as yoga, tai chi, and Pilates can help you improve your range of motion, reduce stiffness and soreness, and prevent injuries.

Cardiovascular exercises:
Cardiovascular exercises such as walking, jogging, cycling, and swimming can help you improve your heart health, reduce your risk of chronic diseases, and maintain a healthy weight.

Walking:

Walking is a low-impact exercise that can help you improve your cardiovascular health, strengthen your bones, and reduce your risk of chronic diseases.

Swimming:

Swimming is a low-impact exercise that can help you build muscle mass, improve your flexibility, and reduce your risk of chronic diseases.

Cycling:

Cycling is a low-impact exercise that can help you improve your cardiovascular health, build muscle mass, and reduce your risk of chronic diseases.

Yoga:

Yoga is a low-impact exercise that can help you improve your flexibility, reduce stress levels, and improve your overall well-being.

Hack 8 – Track Your Food Intake

Tracking food intake can be an effective tool for weight loss. One of the primary ways that tracking food intake can help with weight loss is by increasing awareness of what is being consumed. By keeping track of what is being eaten, individuals can identify areas where they can make healthier choices and reduce their overall calorie intake. Additionally, tracking food intake can help to identify patterns of overeating or unhealthy eating habits, which can be addressed and corrected.

Another way that tracking food intake can help with weight loss is by promoting accountability. When individuals track their food intake, they are more likely to stick to their weight loss goals and make healthier choices. Additionally, tracking food intake can help to prevent mindless eating, which can lead to overeating and weight gain.

Tracking food intake can also help to identify triggers for overeating or unhealthy eating habits. By keeping track of what is being eaten and when, individuals can identify patterns of overeating or unhealthy eating habits, such as eating when stressed or bored. Once these triggers are identified, individuals can take steps to address them and make healthier choices.

Finally, tracking food intake can help to identify nutrient deficiencies. When individuals track their food intake, they can identify areas where they may be lacking in certain nutrients, such as protein or fiber. By identifying these deficiencies, individuals can make changes to their diet to ensure that they are getting the nutrients they need to support weight loss and overall health.

In conclusion, tracking food intake can be an effective tool for weight loss. By increasing awareness of what is being consumed, promoting accountability, identifying triggers for overeating or unhealthy eating habits, and identifying nutrient deficiencies, tracking food intake can help individuals achieve and maintain a healthy weight.

Here are some ideas to help with tracking your food intake:

Use a food diary:

A food diary is a written record of everything you eat and drink. You can use a notebook, a smartphone app, or a website to keep track of your food intake. This can help you identify patterns in your eating habits and make changes to your diet accordingly.

Read food labels:

Food labels tell you how many calories, nutrients, and ingredients are in a food. Reading food labels can help you make informed decisions about what to eat and how much to eat.

Use a calorie-tracking app:

Calorie-tracking apps such as MyFitnessPal, Lose It!, and FatSecret can help you track your food intake, monitor your calorie intake, and set goals for weight loss or weight gain.

Consult a registered dietitian:

A registered dietitian can help you develop a personalized meal plan, track your food intake, and provide guidance on healthy eating habits.

Take photos of your meals:

Taking photos of your meals can help you keep track of what you eat and make healthier choices. You can use your smartphone to take photos of your meals and review them later.

Hack 9 – Eat More Slowly

Eating slowly can be an effective tool for weight loss. One of the primary ways that eating slowly can help with weight loss is by increasing feelings of fullness and reducing hunger. Eating slowly promotes thorough chewing. To eat slowly, you need to chew your food thoroughly before swallowing. This can help you reduce calorie intake and lose weight. In fact, studies show that people who eat slowly tend to be leaner than those who eat quickly. Eating slowly can also help to decrease the amount of food consumed during the meal due to an increase in fullness hormones. In one study, 17 healthy people with a normal weight ate 10.5 ounces (300 grams) of ice cream on 2 occasions. During the first, they at the ice cream within 5 minutes, but during the second, they took 30 minutes. Their reported fullness and levels of fullness hormones increased significantly more after eating the ice cream slowly.

Eating slowly can also help to decrease calorie intake. In one study, people with normal weight or overweight ate at different paces. Both groups ate fewer calories during the slowest-paced meal, although the difference was only statistically significant in the normal-weight group. All participants also felt fuller for longer after eating more slowly, reporting less hunger 60 minutes after the slow meal than after the fast one.

Eating slowly can also help to reduce the number of calories that are absorbed by the body. When food is eaten quickly, it is not properly chewed, which can lead to larger food particles entering the digestive system. This can make it more difficult for the body to absorb nutrients from the food, which can lead to weight gain. By eating slowly and chewing food thoroughly, individuals can help to ensure that food is properly digested and nutrients are properly absorbed.

Finally, eating slowly can help to reduce stress levels. Stress can lead to overeating and weight gain, as well as other health problems such as diabetes and heart disease. By eating slowly and taking time to enjoy meals, individuals can reduce stress levels and promote weight loss.

In conclusion, eating slowly can be an effective tool for weight loss. By increasing feelings of fullness, decreasing calorie intake, reducing the number of calories absorbed by the body, and reducing stress levels, eating slowly can help individuals achieve and maintain a healthy weight.

Here are some ideas to help with eating more slowly:

Put down your utensils between bites:
   Putting down your utensils between bites can help you slow down your eating pace and savor your food.

Chew your food thoroughly:
   Chewing your food thoroughly can help you digest your food better and reduce the risk of choking.

Drink water before and during meals:
   Drinking water before and during meals can help you feel fuller and reduce your calorie intake.

Take breaks during meals:

Taking breaks during meals can help you slow down your eating pace and give your body time to register fullness.

Eat with others:

Eating with others can help you slow down your eating pace and enjoy your food more.

Avoid multitasking while eating:

Avoiding multitasking while eating can help you focus on your food and enjoy it more.

Hack 10 – Find A Support System

Having a support system can be an effective tool for weight loss. One of the primary ways that having a support system can help with weight loss is by providing accountability. When individuals have a support system, they are more likely to stick to their weight loss goals and make healthier choices. Additionally, having a support system can help to provide motivation and encouragement, which can help individuals stay on track with their weight loss goals.

Another way that having a support system can help with weight loss is by providing guidance and support. When individuals have a support system, they have access to a network of people who can provide advice and support when needed. This can be especially helpful when individuals are struggling with weight loss or are facing challenges that they are unsure how to overcome.

Having a support system can also help to provide emotional support. Weight loss can be a difficult and emotional journey, and having a support system can help individuals to cope with the emotional challenges that come with weight loss. Emotional support can help individuals to stay motivated and focused on their weight loss goals, even when faced with setbacks or challenges.

Finally, having a support system can help to provide practical support. Practical support can include things like meal planning, grocery shopping, and exercise partners. By having access to practical support, individuals can make healthier choices and stay on track with their weight loss goals.

In conclusion, having a support system can be an effective tool for weight loss. By providing accountability, guidance and support, emotional support, and practical support, having a support system can help individuals achieve and maintain a healthy weight.

Here are some ideas to help with developing a support system:

Join a weight loss group:

Joining a weight loss group can provide you with a sense of community and support. You can find weight loss groups online or in your local area.

Find a workout buddy:

Finding a workout buddy can help you stay motivated and accountable. You can find a workout buddy through social media, online forums, or your local gym.

Enlist the help of a personal trainer:

A personal trainer can help you develop a personalized workout plan, track your progress, and provide guidance on healthy eating habits.

Use a weight loss app:

Weight loss apps such as MyFitnessPal, Lose It!, and FatSecret can help you track your food intake, monitor your calorie intake, and set goals for weight loss or weight gain.

Talk to your friends and family:

Talking to your friends and family about your weight loss goals can help you stay motivated and accountable. They can provide you with emotional support and encouragement.

Conclusion

osing weight can be a challenging process, especially for men aged over 40. However, by making small changes to your lifestyle, you can achieve significant results. For example, drinking more water, eating slowly, and getting enough sleep can help you reduce your calorie intake and improve your digestion. Choosing whole foods, strength training, and reducing sugar intake can help you maintain a healthy diet and build muscle mass. Using a calorie-tracking app, joining a weight loss group, and practicing relaxation techniques can help you stay motivated and accountable.

Remember, the key to successful weight loss is consistency and persistence. By incorporating these weight loss hacks into your daily routine, you can achieve your goals and maintain a healthy lifestyle.

Good luck on your weight loss journey!